Dedication

I dedicate this journal to my friend, Debbie Kelly. You have chosen a career to help pregnant women succeed in their journey of motherhood. It is a special time in a woman's life. A season of life that is encountered with joy and enthusiasm but also uncertainty and often fear of the unknown. May God bless you abundantly and may he shower you with endless blessings.

María A Flores

THE LORD IS MY

Light

AND

Salvation

PSALM 27:1

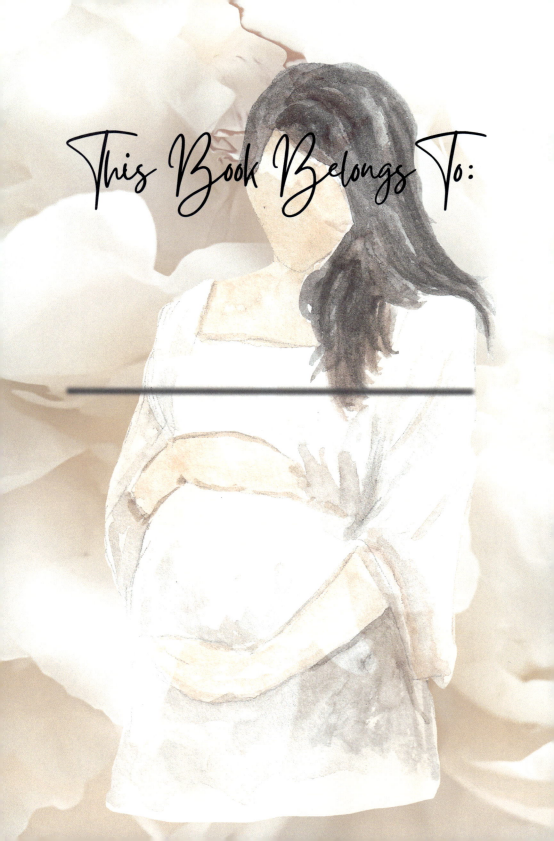

This Book Belongs To:

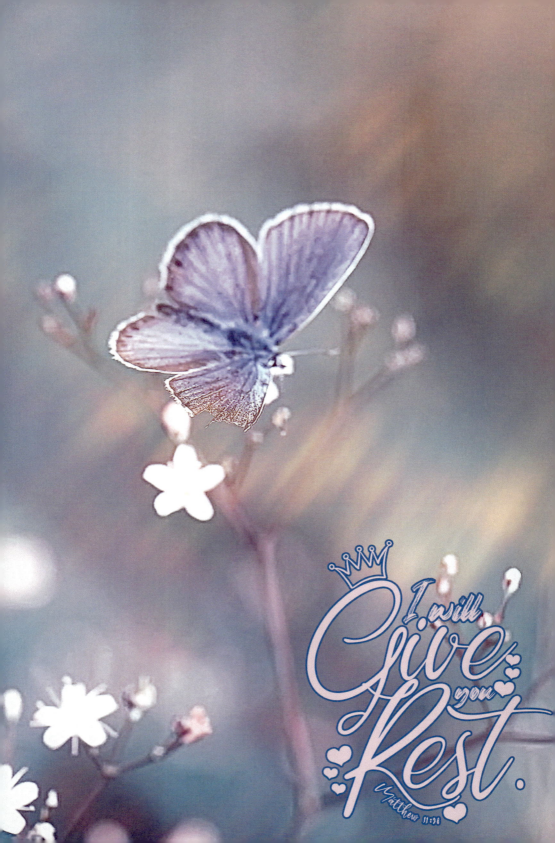

I will
Give
you
Rest.

Matthew 11:28

Prayer Book for Expecting Mothers

A Journey of Courage & Love

By: Maria A Flores

Prayer Book for Expecting Mothers: A Journey of Courage and Love

Touch the Heart, Reach the Soul LLC
Author, Illustrator, Book Cover Designer:
Maria A Flores

Scripture quotations are from the ESV Bible (The Holy Bible, English Standard Version), 2001 by Crossway, a publishing ministry of Good News Publishers. Used by Permission. All rights reserved.

The pictures of people in this book were computer generated.

Inspirational faith based books, journals, planners, notebooks, apparel, jewelry and gift items.

http://touchtheheartreachthesoul.store
touchtheheart.customerservice@gmail.com

Contents

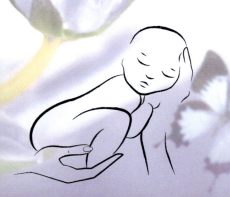

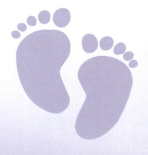

Chapter 1

My Sheep Hear my Voice

"I am the good shepherd. I know my own and my own know me, just as the Father knows me and I know the Father; and I lay down my life for the sheep. And I have other sheep that are not of this fold. I must bring them also, and they will listen to my voice. So there will be one flock, one shepherd. For this reason the Father loves me, because I lay down my life that I may take it up again."
(John 10:14-17)

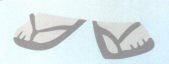

A Message of Love

"Do not fear daughter of God. I will meet your needs and your infant's needs. Place your faith in me.

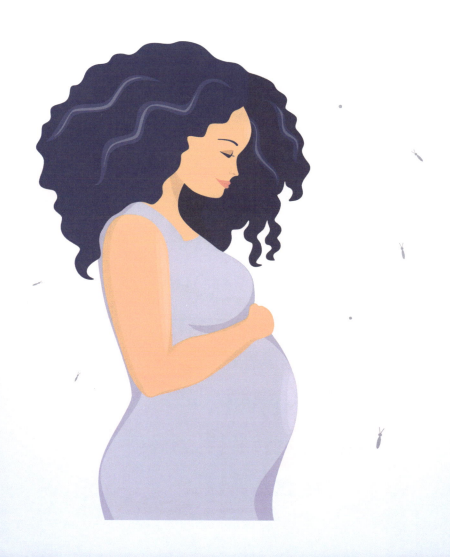

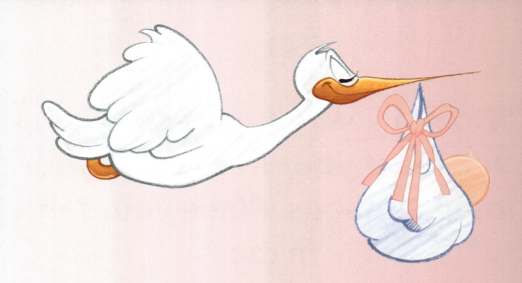

I AM your provider. Your child is my blessing to you. Love your child. You will smile, you will cry but know you are not alone.
It is through hardships that you will discover your strength is through ME.

In ME,
through ME and
with ME.

This is how you are to live your life:

Abide in my love, my safety, my will, my protection, my guidance.
Abide in Me daughter.
You are my precious beloved daughter.

Do not listen to the lies of the enemy.

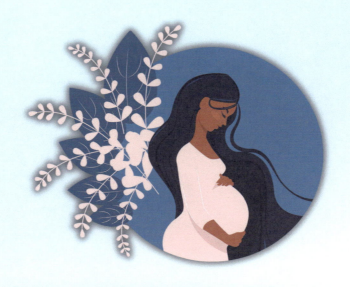

I have not told you any of
these things yet you hold them
close to your heart.

You are worthy.
You are lovely.
You are beautiful.
You are more than enough.
You were wonderfully made in
MY IMAGE.

LISTEN TO ME.

Since the day you were born
I loved you unconditionally.
Do not look at your
circumstances or your belly
with hatred instead look at
me.
I AM with you.

Father
Son
Holy Spirit

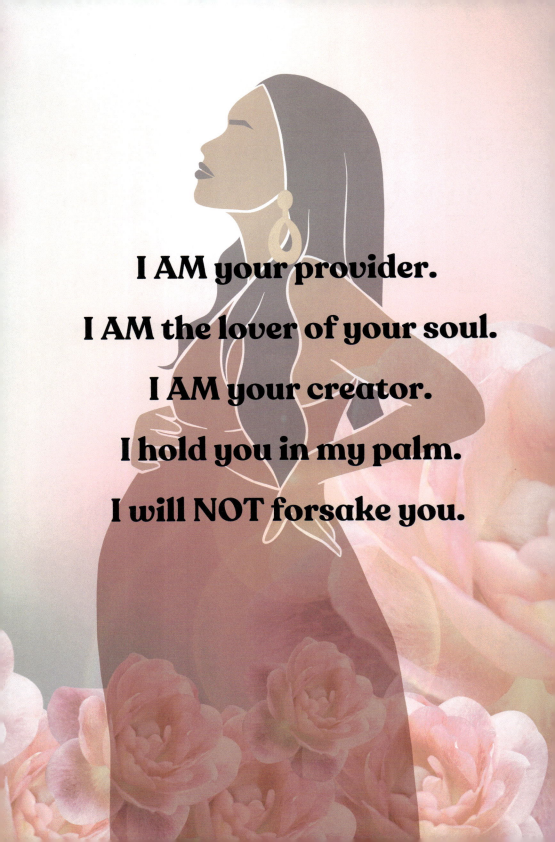

I AM your provider.

I AM the lover of your soul.

I AM your creator.

I hold you in my palm.

I will NOT forsake you.

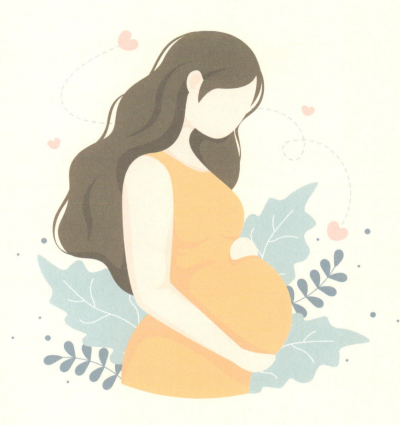

Allow me into your life. I will show you what true love is. I AM love.
Get to know my son, JESUS. He died for you. Through Him, you will find Me. I AM the great I AM."

Prayer

May your tears of grief turn into tears of joy.
May your heavy heart be filled with lovely thoughts of what is to come.
May your child light up your heart with joy.
May you discover the love of Christ.

Maria A Flores

Prayer Requests

Date

Chapter 2

Created Out of Love

You were created by your Heavenly Father out of love. In His image, you were made. You were given free will. You can choose to partake in His great love by making Jesus your Lord and Savior.

Do not be fooled by what the world says regarding gods. There is one Holy, Magestic Creator and there is only one way to reach His presence and experience His great love for you.

Ask God to manifest himself to you. He will often manifest himself during prayer, worship and when reading the Holy Bible.

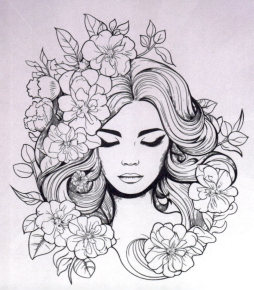

Love

For God so loved the world that he gave His only begotten Son, that whosoever believeth in Him shall not perish, but have everlasting life.
(John 3:16)

Jesus saith onto to him, I am the way, the truth and the life: no man cometh unto the Father, but by me.
(John 14:16)

Let all that you do be done in love.
(1 Corinthians 16:14)

Greater love has no one than this, that someone lay down his life for his friend.
(John 15:13)

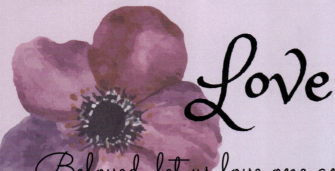

Love

Beloved, let us love one another, for love is of God and whoever loves has been born of God and knows God.
(1 John 4:7)

As the Father has loved me, so have I loved you. Abide in my love. If you keep my commandments, you will abide in my love, just as I have kept my Father's commandments and abide in his love.
(John 15: 9-10)

"You shall love the Lord your God with all of your heart and with all of your soul and with all of your mind. This is the great and first commandment.
(Matthew 22:36)

Prayer to Receive Love

Heavenly Father:
Help me to receive your perfect love. Help me to forgive myself and others that have hurt me. I want to have a relationship with you and I accept you as my father. I receive your love now.

Amen

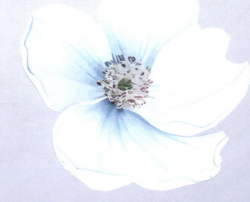

Self Declarations

I am God's beloved daughter.
I am deeply loved by my creator.
I am a child of the most High God.
I extend my love to others freely.
I am able to love myself and my baby.
I will love others and be kind to those around me.

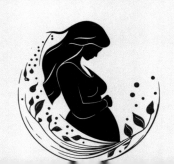

Declarations for Baby

My baby is wanted and loved.
My baby is deeply loved by our creator.
My child has a Heavenly Father.
Angels have been assigned to protect my baby.
My child will experience the love of God.
My baby is blessed in all aspects of life.

Prayer Requests

Date

_____

_____

_____

_____

_____

_____

_____

_____

_____

_____

_____

_____

_____

Chapter 3

Created with a Purpose

You have a purpose, mission and calling upon your life. It is not by chance you are reading this book.

The choice is yours.

If you choose the narrow and righteous path, you are guaranteed eternal glory and salvation. The journey will still be challenging, however you no longer carry the load alone. Now you have a partner for life (God, Jesus and the Holy Spirit) whom will guide you and protect you.

The choice is yours.

Decide who you will serve. You cannot serve other gods for God is a jealous God and requests that believers keep the first commandment. Will you choose a life of freedom, joy everlasting and abounding blessings ?

The Greatest Commandment

And you shall love the Lord your God with all your heart and with all your soul and with all your mind and with all your strength.
(Mark 12:30)

No one can serve two masters, for either he will hate one, and love the other, or he will be devoted to the one and despise the other. You cannot serve God and money..
(Matthew 6:24)

So we have come to know and to believe the love that God has for us. God is love, and whoever abides in love abides in God, and God abides in him.
(1 John 4:16)

Life Everlasting

...then the Lord God formed the man of dust from the ground and breathed into his nostrils the breath of life, and the man became a living creature. (Genesis 1:30)

"Truly, truly, I say to you. Whoever believes has eternal life."
(John 6:47)

"See, I have set before you today life and good, death and evil."
(Deuteronomy 28:66)

Whoever believes in the Son has eternal life, whoever does not obey the Son shall not see life, but the wrath of God remains in him.
(John 3:36)

Prayer to Discover my Purpose in Life

Dear Father:

You created me out of love with a purpose and an assignment to fulfill. Holy Spirit, you are welcomed into my life. Guide me in every step of my journey. Close doors that need to close and open doors that will allow me to prosper in my life.

Self Declarations

I was created with a purpose, mission and calling upon my life.
I will discover my purpose.
I will allow the Holy Spirit to guide me into my divine journey.
I will proceed with caution and follow the narrow path.
I know that fear is from the enemy, therefore I walk with courage towards my future.
I will keep my eyes on you, Lord.

Declarations for Baby

My baby was created to join the great kingdom of God.

As my child grows, he/she will find their true destiny of life.

My child will encounter the love of Christ.

My child is set apart, chosen to do great things and will be a blessing to those around him/her.

My child will prosper and live a life of peace, joy and happiness.

Prayer Requests

Date

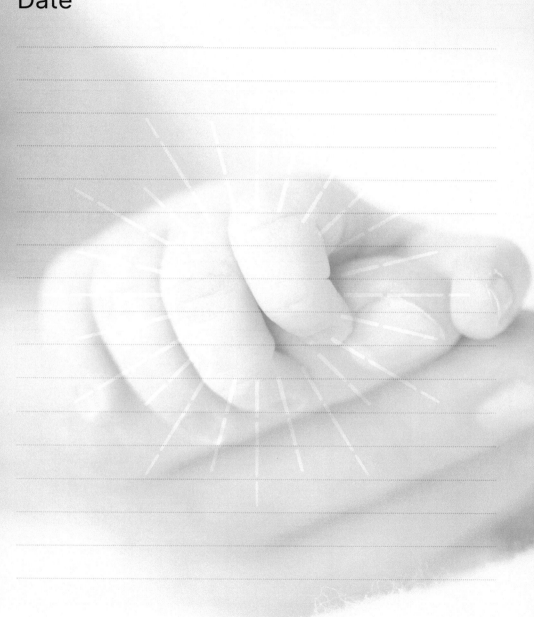

Chapter 4

Walking by Faith

On a personal note, my husband and I spent 5 years unable to conceive. But God, had a different plan for us and children were part of His blessing. We spent those years seeking God's face, praying fervently and walking in faith for the dream that one day we would have a family. One day, we were blessed with a daughter and later two sons.

Faith is believing in the unseen with our natural eyes. This can be for a current situation or for a future event.

God gives us a vision before He gives us provision. The Lord tells us in the Holy Bible, to seek Him and to ask Him with our petitions. Stand in faith and wait upon the Lord until you see the manifestation of your miracle!

Living by Faith

But without faith it is impossible to please him, for whoever would draw near to God must believe that he exists and that he rewards those who seek him.
(Hebrews 11:6)

Now faith is the assurance of things hoped for, the conviction of things not seen.
(Hebrews 11:1)

"If anyone would come after me, let him deny himself and take up his cross daily and follow me. For whoever would save his life will lose it, but whoever loses his life for my sake will save it. For what does it profit a man if he gains the whole world and loses or forfeits himself?"
(Luke 9:23-24)

Pray, Believe, Receive

"If you have faith as a grain of mustard seed ... nothing shall be impossible unto you."
(Matthew 17:20)

"Therefore I tell you, whatever you ask in prayer, believe that you have received it, and it will be yours."
(Mark 11:24)

For we walk by faith, not by sight.
(1 Corinthians 5:7)

Because you have made the Lord your dwelling place - the most High, who is my refuge - no evil shall be allowed to befall you, no plague come near your tent. For he will command his angels concerning you to guard you in all your ways.
(Psalm 91:9-14)

Prayer to Increase Faith

Dear Jesus:

I pray that my faith will increase as I go through this season of my life. I believe in your promises of blessings upon my life. Help me to stay committed to following you and acknowledge you in all of my decisions for the rest of my life.

Amen

Self Declarations

I walk by faith.
I will continue to be faithful even during difficult times.
To increase my faith, I will hear and read the word of God daily.
I have faith God will meet my needs.
I am rooted in Christ and unshakable.
My words are powerful, therefore I use my words wisely and instill faith in those around me.

Declarations for Baby

My baby will be born healthy.
My baby will have more than
enough to meet his/her needs.
My child will be favored in all
situations.
My baby will be the head and
not the tail.
My baby is shielded from the
attacks of the enemy (in the
womb and once he/she is
born).
My baby will grow up to be a
courageous man/woman of
God.

Prayer Requests

Date

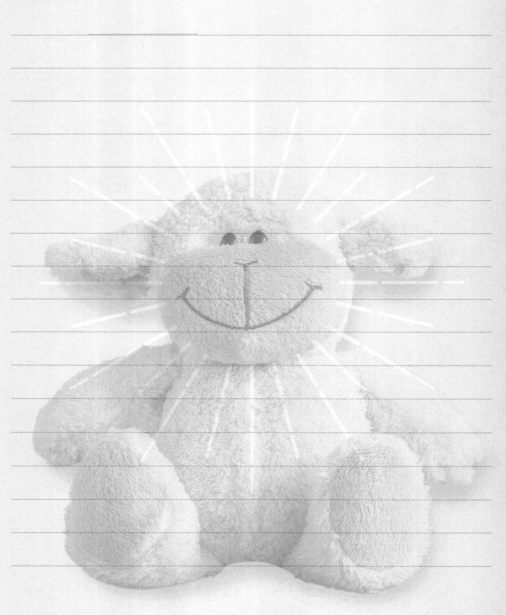

Chapter 5

Follow The Narrow Path

We were created with free will. Therefore, each person has the ability to make decisions every day on how he/she will live. Every decision we make has a consequence. We can choose to live a righteous life, which will lead us to prosperity or we can make poor decisions, which will lead to negative consequences.

When we make the decision to follow Jesus, it is indeed the 'narrow path.' It is the harder path, the one with more challenges. Jesus refers to His sheep as his followers. The Father knows who His true followers are. He knows our most inner, deepest thoughts. After all, He formed us in our mother's womb. When you call upon the name of the Lord, He will hear you and help you in times of need. Commit your life to the Lord and He will direct your path into holiness. This will result in increased peace, joy, protection and abundance of blessings.

One Path to Salvation

For unto you is born this day in the city of David a Savior, who is Christ the Lord.
(Luke 2:11)

For by grace you have been saved through faith. And this is not your own doing; it is the gift of God, not a result of works, so that no one may boast.
(Ephesians 2:8)

For the wages of sin is death, but the free gift of God is eternal life in Christ Jesus our Lord.
(Romans 6:23)

I AM the Truth

And there is salvation in on one else, for there is no other name under heaven given among men by which we must be saved. (Acts 4:12)

...Because greater is He that is in you, than he that is in the world. (1 John 4:4)

And we have seen and testify that the Father has sent his Son to be the Savior of the world. (1 John 4:14)

Prayer to Follow Jesus

Dear Jesus:

Help me to follow the narrow path. Show me the way towards my destiny. Help me to abide in your dwelling and remain in your presence.

Forgive me for my sins. Bring me back into your dwelling and secret place of protection.

Self Declarations

I follow the narrow path.
I keep my mind on God.
I will not be shaken.
I keep my priorities in the right order: God, Family, Work
I will focus on God's glory and His kingdom.
I was born for such a time as this.
I am the leader of the flock.
I shall rise as high as an eagle.
I am not transformed by the things of this world but rather commissioned to fulfill my glory assignment.

Declarations for Baby

My child will follow the narrow path.

My child will grow up to be an honorable man or woman of God.

True identity is found in Christ.

My child has favor amongst his or her peers.

My child will discover the purpose of life and fulfill the calling upon his/her life in due time.

Prayer Requests

Date

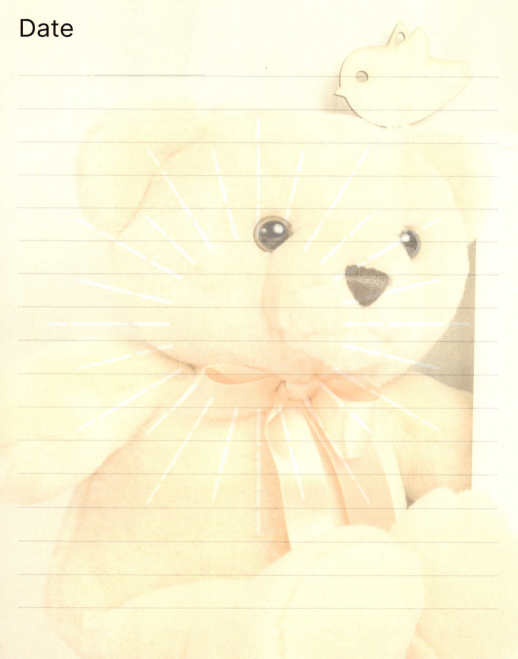

Chapter 6

Your Assignment

We each have an assignment to fulfill within the body of Christ. You have God given unique gifts and talents. Take a closer look at your life and reflect on the areas you are naturally good at. Your gift may be in speaking, creative art, writing or something else. Use your gifts to glorify God and He will bless you abundantly.

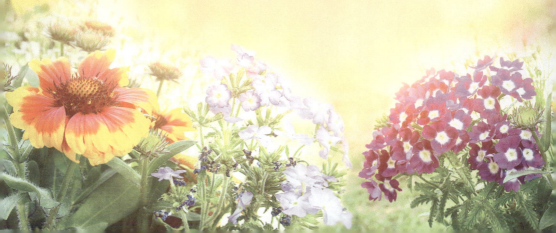

God Speaks to his People

(God speaking to Moses)
"I am the God of your fathers, the God of Abraham, Isaac and Jacob."
(Acts 7:32)

Draw nigh (close) to God, and he will draw nigh to you.
(James 4:8)

He that dwelleth in the secret place of the most High shall abide under the shadow of the almighty.
(Psalm 91:1)

But the Helper, the Holy Spirit, whom the Father will send in my name, he will teach you all things and bring to your remembrance all that I have said.
(John 14:26)

Discovering Your Purpose

For we are His workmanship, created in Christ Jesus for good works, which God prepared beforehand, that we should walk in them.
(Ephesians 2:10)

Trust in the Lord with all of your heart, and do not lean on your own understanding. In all your ways acknowledge Him, and He will make straight your paths.
(Proverbs 3:5-6)

Before I formed you in the womb I knew you, and before you were born I consecrated you. (Jeremiah 1:5)

For I know the plans I have for you, declares the Lord, plans for welfare and not for evil, to give you a future and hope.
(Jeremiah 29:11)

Prayer to Hear God's Voice

Dear Father:
Help me to hear your voice clearly. Help me to cast down thoughts that are against your will and commandments. I want to serve you and you alone. I glorify and worship you. You are my beloved father. Help me to discern your voice from mine and the enemy. Thank you for hearing my petitions.

Self Declarations

I was made for a time such as this.
I have purpose and meaning in my life.
I recognize the voice of my Heavenly Father.
I will discover my glory assignment and fulfill it with God's help.
I will use my God given gifts and talents to work towards my mission.
I have faith that the necessary tools, people and resources will fall within my path at the right appointed time.

Declarations for Baby

My child has a calling and purpose in the kingdom of God.

My child will discover his/her God given talents and use them to glorify God and to enhance the body of Christ.

My child holds an appointed assignment that will be revealed to him/her at an appointed time and season.

Chapter 7
You are Not Alone

The enemy wants humanity to believe we are alone in life's struggles. In reality, we have the choice to walk on our path alone or to walk alongside Jesus.

If you accept Jesus into your heart as your Lord and Savior, He will equip you with the resources necessary to get through your journey successfully.

Like gold that needs fire to be purified, going through challenges can also make us stronger. Daughter of God, remember, you are not alone.

Walking with Christ

"In the beginning was the Word, and the Word was with God, and the Word was God. (John 1:1)

But you will receive power when the Holy Spirit has come upon you, and you will be my witnesses in Jerusalem... and to the end of the earth. (Acts 1:8)

So faith comes from hearing, and hearing through the word of Christ. (Romans 10:17)

If we confess our sins, He is faithful and just to forgive us our sins and to cleanse us from all unrighteousness. (1 John 1:9)

Take His Hand

Jesus said to him, " I am the way, and the truth, and the life. No one comes to the Father except through me."
(John 14:6)

Then Jesus told his disciples, "If anyone would come after me, let him deny himself and take up his cross and follow me."
(Matthew 16:24)

For with the heart one believes and is justified, and with the mouth one confesses and is saved.
(Rmans 10:10)

" I am the light of the world. Whoever follows me will not walk in darkness, but will have the light of life."
(John 8:12)

Prayer to Abide in Jesus

Jesus: You are my savior. You suffered and died for me. I want to live my life with you by my side. Will you hold my hand as I navigate this life? You have always been there for me. Never let me go and remember me. I proclaim, I am in the book of life and I will enter the gates of heaven. Help me to keep you in my life and stay focused on my mission and glory assignment you have given me. I love you Jesus.

Self Declarations

I clearly hear and recognize the voice of my Heavenly Father.

I refuse to hear the voice of the enemy.

I will cast down all intrusive thoughts that do not align with the word of God.

I will spend time in prayer to maintain my spiritual health.

When the Lord speaks to me, I will take the time to write his message.

My mind, heart and emotions are at peace.

I will not allow discord and unforgiveness to enter my home.

Declarations for Baby

My child will feel the love of Christ.

My child can rest peacefully.

My son/daughter will be safe and secure all the days of his/her life.

My child is a light in the darkness.

My child will tread upon serpents.

He/she will be a great man/woman of God.

Prayer Requests

Date

Chapter 8

Enjoy Your Baby

The enemy wants you to believe that children are a burden and your life as you know it will cease to exist. You will experience a change in your life. The season of your life will change as you transition into motherhood. However, your child will become your greatest miracle and blessing.

New challenges arise but new blessings also are on the horizon. The first time your child smiles at you, kisses you, and laughs are very special moments, like no other. Enjoy your baby!

Seasons of Life

The Lord will open to you his good treasury, the heavens, to give the rain to your land in its season and to bless all the work of your hands. And you shall lend to many nations, but you shall not borrow.
(Deuteronomy 28:12)

To make an apt answer is a joy to a man, and a word in season, how good it is!
(Proverbs 15:23)

The eyes of all look to you, and you give them food in due season.
(Psalm 145:15)

For everything there is a season, and a time for every matter under heaven.
(Ecclesiastes 3:1)

Your Faith will Carry You

The Lord passed before him and proclaimed, "The Lord, a God merciful and gracious, slow to anger, and abounding in steadfast love and faithfulness." (Exodus 34:6)

"And if you faithfully obey the voice of the Lord your God, being careful to do all his commandments that I command you today, the Lord your God will set you high above the nations of the earth." (Deuteronomy 28:1)

"Now therefore fear the Lord and serve him in sincerity and in faithfulness." (Joshua 24:14)

Rejoicing in God's Goodness

Dear Jesus:

Today I want to thank you for all of the blessings in my life. As I wait for the arrival of my baby, I will abide by your steadfast love and promises upon my life. I trust in you and have faith in your words. I will not take anything for granted and recognize all good things come from you. Thank you for giving me one more day to enjoy my life.

Amen

Self Declarations

I have the courage to fulfill my role as a mother.

I realize that loving someone is a conscious decision therefore I am making the decision to love myself and my child.

I will make an effort to maintain peace, harmony and unity in my family.

If I am within a loving and secure relationship with my child's father, I will include him in the role of parenting to enhance stability and foster a stable environment for my baby.

Declarations for Baby

I will teach my baby about the love of Christ.
I will lead by example.
I will be firm but loving in the upbringing of my baby with the understanding that children need clear boundaries to succeed during their childhood.
My child will learn to lean on Jesus.
My baby is abundantly blessed.

Prayer Requests

Date

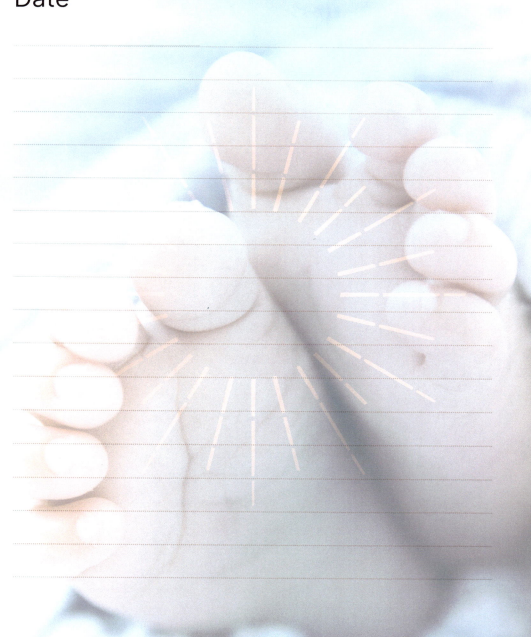

Chapter 9

The Battle

You are in a daily battle. Recognize the enemy wants you to be miserable, suffering, alone and silent. Gain knowledge on how Satan and his followers operate. "Know your enemy." The Christian walk is one of constant spiritual battle. God has given us ways to fight evil. Living a life of prayer is necessary. You will gain wisdom, understanding and knowledge by reading the Bible. Stand In the gap of the ungodly and pray that God will touch the hearts of the unholy causing them to turn from their wickedness to holiness.

The Battlefield

For we do not wrestle against flesh and blood, but against the rulers, against the authorities, against the cosmic powers over this present darkness, against the spiritual forces of evil in the heavenly places. (Ephesians 6:12)

Submit yourselves therefore to God. Resist the devil, and he will feel from you. (James 4:7)

And that all this assembly may know that the Lord saves not with the sword and spear. For the battle is the Lord's, and he will give you into our hand. (1 Samuel 17:47)

And no wonder, for even Satan disguises himself as an angel of light. (2 Corinthians 11:14)

Understand Your Opponent

... the prince of the power of the air, the spirit that is now at work in the sons of disobedience— among whom we all once lived in the passions of our flesh, carrying out the desires of the body and mind... But God, being rich in mercy, because of the great love with which he loved us, made us alive together with Christ— by grace you have been saved.
(Ephesians 2:2-4

Submit yoursleves therefore to God. Resist the devil, and he will flee from you. Draw near to God, and he will draw near to you.
(James 4:8)

The reason the Son of God appeared was to destroy the works of the devil... By this it is evident who are the children of God, and who are the children of the devil.
(1 John 3:8-10)

Prayer to Gain Wisdom

Jesus: You are my savior. You suffered and died for me. I want to live my life with you by my side. Will you hold my hand as I navigate this life? You have always been there for me. Never let me go and remember me. I proclaim, I am in the book of life and I will enter the gates of heaven. Help me to keep you in my life and stay focused on my mission and glory assignment you have given me. I love you Jesus.

Self Declarations

I clearly hear and recognize the voice of my Heavenly Father.

I refuse to hear the voice of the enemy.

I will cast down all intrusive through ts that do not align with the word of God.

I will spend time in prayer to maintain my spiritual health.

When the Lord speaks to me, I will take the time to write his message.

My mind, heart and emotions are at peace.

I will not allow discord and unforgiveness to enter my home.

Declarations for Baby

My child will feel the love of Christ.

My child can rest peacefully.

My son/daughter will be safe and secure all the days of his/her life.

My child is a light in the darkness.

My child will tread upon serpents.

He/she will be a great man/woman of God.

Prayer Requests

Date

Chapter 10
Put on the Armor of God

People often wonder why do bad things happen to good people? Although this can be difficult to answer, most Christians would agree that people are vulnerable to attacks when they are unprotected from the hand of God. In other words, they lack a spiritual covering.

God has given us the tools to protect ourselves from the enemy. It is up to us to use them and fight back when the enemy attacks. We are not promised a life free from pain, challenges or discomfort. It is often through these challenges, that we grow as human beings as well as learn to rely on Him for our needs.

We are promised eternal life with Jesus if we follow His teachings, believe He is our Lord and Savior and walk a life of righteousness by His side.

The Armor of God

Therefore take up the whole armor of God, that you may be able to withstand in the evil day, and stand firm. Stand therefore, having fastened on the belt of truth, and having put on the breastplate of righteousness, and, as shoes for your feet, having put on the readiness given by the gospel of peace.
(Ephesians, 6:13-15)

In all circumstances, take up the shield of faith, with which you can extinguish all the flaming darts of the evil one and take the helmet of salvation, and the sword of the Spirit, which is the word of God, praying at all times in the Spirit, with all prayer and supplication.
(Ephesians 6: 16-17)

For though we walk in flesh, we are not waging war according to the flesh.
(2 Corinthians 10:3)

Remain Watchful

No weapon that is formed against you shall succeed, and you shall refute every tongue that rises against you in judgement.
(Isaiah 54:17)

For the Lord God is a sun and shield; the Lord bestows favor and honor. No good thing does He withhold from those who walk upright.
(Psalm 84:11)

Truly, I say to you, whatever you bind on earth shall be bound in heaven, and whatever you loose on earth shall be loosed in heaven.
(Matthew 18:18-20)

And you will know the truth, and the truth shall set you free.
(John 8:32)

Prayer for Courage

Dear Beloved Jesus:
I ask you to give me the courage to fight the good fight. Help me to remain strong and steadfast in your love and security. Renew my strength in you daily. I ask you to give me a spirit of courage, fierce fullness, righteousness, audacity, and a sound mind. Help me to fight for my family every day of my life. I stand ready for the battle. I am your warrior.

Self Declarations

I declare I am prayer warrior.
I will fight for myself and my
family daily.
I will maintain the unity of my
family.
I allow the Holy Spirit to guide me
in every step of the battle.
I am not afraid of challenges and
difficult times, for God is with me.
I will be a good role model for my
children.
I will be relentless in my pursuit to
complete my glory assignment.
I will fulfill all that God has
assigned for me to complete on
this earth.

Declarations for Baby

My child is the head and not the tail.

I place a ring of Holy Spirit fire around my child and no weapon of the enemy shall penetrate.

My child will also become a warrior of Christ.

My son/daughter will live life courageously.

He/she will experience an abundance of love and never doubt God's presence, mercy and grace.

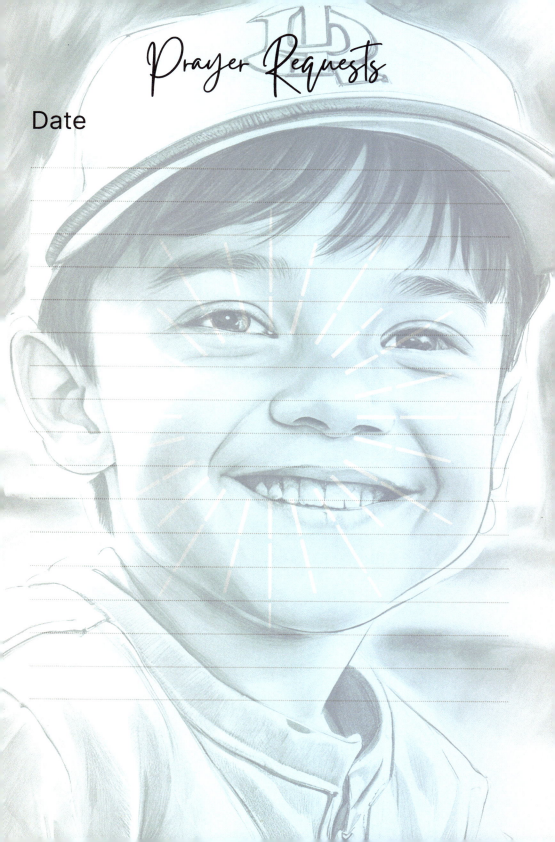

Prayer Requests

Date

About the Author

Maria Flores is a wife, mother, nurse, and writer. She is the founder of Touch the Heart, Reach the Soul. The mission of this organization is to increase the intimacy of people to God through Christian inspirational books, jewelry and apparel. She believes individuals can find joy and freedom once they discover the purpose, calling, and mission God has placed upon their lives. She currently resides in Florida with her husband and children.

Journals & Books

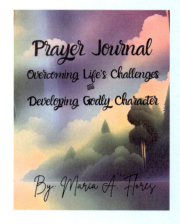

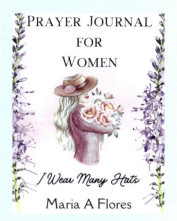

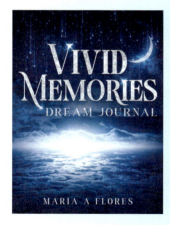

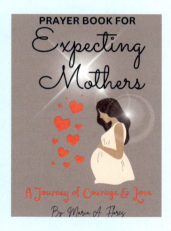

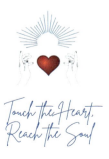

Touch the Heart, Reach the Soul

Coloring Books

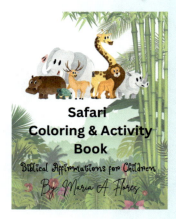

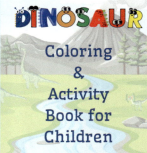

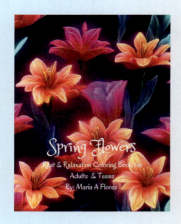

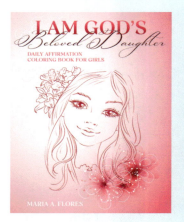

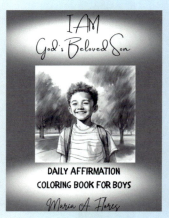

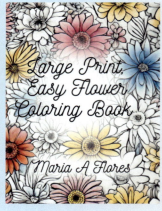

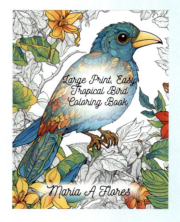

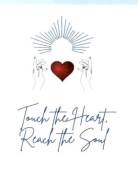

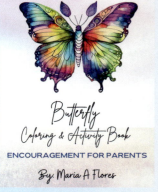

Notebooks

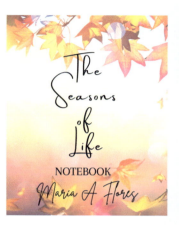

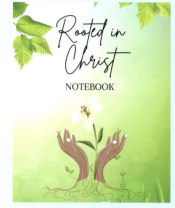

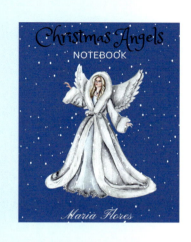

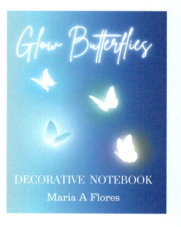

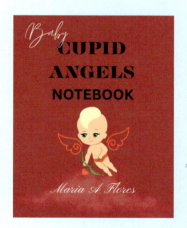

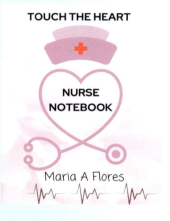

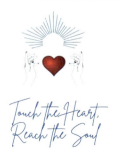

Planners

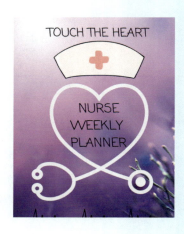

TOUCH THE HEART

NURSE WEEKLY PLANNER

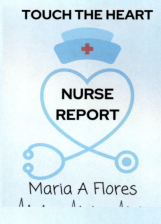

TOUCH THE HEART

NURSE REPORT

Maria A Flores

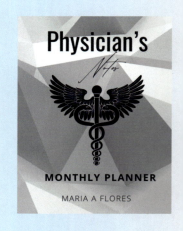

Physician's Notes

MONTHLY PLANNER

MARIA A FLORES

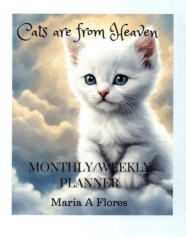

Cats are from Heaven

MONTHLY/WEEKLY PLANNER

Maria A Flores

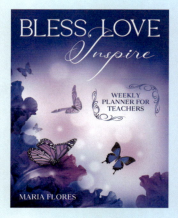

BLESS, LOVE Inspire

WEEKLY PLANNER FOR TEACHERS

MARIA FLORES

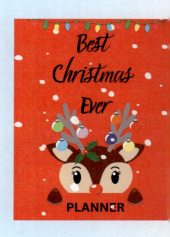

Best Christmas Ever

PLANNER

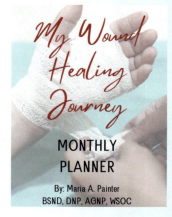

My Wound Healing Journey

MONTHLY PLANNER

By: Maria A. Painter
BSND, DNP, AGNP, WSOC

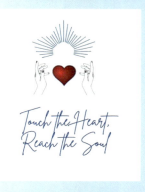

Touch the Heart, Reach the Soul